THE ABCs OF MAKING IT IN THE ED

A guide to becoming an asset in the emergency department for medical students, nurse practitioners, physician assistants, and resident physicians

Jason A. Borton, M.D.

DEDICATION

This book is dedicated to the emergency medicine physicians who have served as thoughtful and dedicated mentors along my road to becoming an attending physician. My second wish of thanks goes out to the nurses who give their best each time they walk into the emergency department. Last, but not least, I thank my patients who keep me interested in the profession and teach me something new every shift.

ACKNOWLEDGEMENTS

I wish to thank John McNamara, M.D, Katie Miller, PA, and Christine Verni, DNP for their time and insightful and heartfelt criticisms that they provided in reviewing this work.

CONTENTS

CHAPTER 1
I'M YOUR CAPTAIN

Hello, it's me, your friendly captain. I'm the commander of the ship we call the emergency department, or the ED, or less correctly, the ER. We're going to be working together for a while, so make it a point during your first shift to approach me and introduce yourself. Tell me your full name and tell me your position. Nothing bothers me more than someone who presents two or three patients to me and then decides to introduce himself. You're going to be introducing yourself to patients, so why not practice your greeting with me first? I have the power to make your time in the department a great learning experience or to make it completely miserable. Let's start off on a good note.

I may repeat your name if I am unsure of the pronunciation. Please correct me if I'm saying your name incorrectly. I'll be mentioning your name to your patients and the nurses throughout the shift and I want to say it correctly.

If you are an emergency medicine resident and I haven't seen you in months, don't expect me to remember your name. Please briefly reintroduce yourself. If I pass you in a hallway and I've only met you once or twice, don't be surprised when my head turns sideways like a dog hearing a high pitched unfamiliar sound when you say "Hi" like we're best friends. I'm lucky that I can remember where to find my car in the doctors' parking lot, much less remember your name.

If you're a physician assistant or a nurse practitioner and we will be working together often, please don't introduce yourself at the beginning of every shift. A simple "Good morning" or "I got you a coffee" will suffice. Do find out what I like to be called. In front of patients, I like to be addressed as Dr. Borton, but I feel weird being addressed as that by a co-worker of fifteen years. If there's a question, please ask me or your preceptor.

CHAPTER 2
YOU'RE ONLY HUMAN

I f we're working together, there's only so much history, physical, and abnormal lab values that we can talk about until I'll become utterly bored and grumpy. I have worked thousands of hours over many years. I am confident that I have untreated ADHD and that's why I chose emergency medicine as a career. If we're going to be working together for a month, a year, or a career, I want to know something about you besides being a provider in the ED.

I might ask you about past careers or where you are from. If you tell me about a hobby or passion of yours that I find interesting, expect me to ask you for more information. By nature, most of us are social beings and by asking you about your likes outside of work, it's my way of saying "I think you're interesting beyond your ability to provide emergency medical care."

I missed these hints from attending physicians as a medical student and a resident physician. I was all business when learning about medicine. I didn't take time to listen to attending's stories. I didn't socialize with my fellow residents. You will find that some attendings are strictly business when they work a shift in the ED. Don't take personal offense. They are probably like that with everyone. They may become more relaxed in future shifts with you. Your attending physician and co-workers should be able to get a feel for what kind of a person you are. It should be realized that not everyone is a social butterfly. On the other end of things, an emergency department can get notoriously busy and stressful. Some people can talk all day if they are permitted to do so. If you have work to do, politely tell them that you're swamped, but that you can talk to them later.

It is important to realize that some employees in the emergency department may prod you for information that you are not comfortable divulging. You should never have to endure any harassment in the work environment. If it occurs, firmly tell the offender that it must stop immediately. If it does not, take a written report of the events that occurred to that person's supervisor.

CHAPTER 3
I'M SINKING QUICKLY SIR

I have met many medical students who appropriately introduce themselves to me right off the bat when they are
rotating in the emergency department. That introduction
is almost always followed up with the question of whether or
not it is kosher for them to pick up a new patient without my
pre-screening of the case. I suspect that many of my attending colleagues are rightfully keeping a watchful eye on the
students, but I always encourage my students and residents
to go into the room and see the patient. I do add the caveat
that if they walk in and they are concerned that the patient
is not looking well or seems to be experiencing a life-threatening event, that they come and get me immediately.

As any level of practitioner, it is vitally important that
you learn to recognize immediate threats to a patient's life.
This is done by addressing the ABCs. A stands for airway.
If a patient can't speak or seems to have a significant injury
or condition that hinders the adequate movement of air
into the lungs, then the airway problem must be corrected

immediately. B is for breathing problems. They can be treated many ways depending on the cause of the problem, but they must be addressed quickly. C is for circulation. A person with a symptomatically low blood pressure has a circulation problem, as does the patient who is bleeding profusely from a wound. These problems need decisive and rapid attention.

When you are in the ED, go into rooms where people are being resuscitated. Learn to recognize what a truly sick patient looks like. One would think that this would come naturally, especially for seasoned physicians, but I've seen several instances where patients would have been helped more by having a housekeeper in the room. A cardiologist that kept talking to an unresponsive and pulseless patient in ventricular tachycardia still haunts my dreams. Luckily, an alert nurse was passing the room and got help. The patient was defibrillated back into giving his history to the cardiologist. Learn to recognize a sick patient and when you need additional help for the patient.

CHAPTER 4
TAKE A SEAT

Now it's time for you to go see your patient. Double check the room number, the patient's name, their vital signs, and the chief complaint. When you arrive at the threshold, make your imminent entrance known by some means. An audible knock and asking to come in will usually work. Wait for an answer. Outside a curtained area, briefly introduce yourself and ask if it is OK to enter the room. Patients get caught up in potentially embarrassing situations in the ED, from not being able to figure out how to put on a hospital gown to having to use a bedside commode or a bedpan at an inopportune moment. Make sure to respect their privacy.

When you do enter the room, introduce yourself and tell the patient your title and that you plan to interview them and perform a physical exam. If the patient refuses to be examined, ask them what their concerns are as you may be able to quell their fears. If they still refuse, politely excuse yourself from the room and speak to your attending physician immediately.

If your patient has stable vital signs and appears somewhat comfortable, pull up a seat and sit down when interviewing them. Research has shown that patients perceive that their provider is spending a great deal of time with them if the provider sits down when obtaining the history. Of course, if the patient is in obvious distress or has issues with his airway, breathing, or circulation, do not sit down. In this case, it is important for you to address their immediate needs by getting your attending physician into the room. As you mature in your practice of emergency medicine, you will become more comfortable with addressing these needs by yourself.

If a patient has a suspected kidney stone, I will enter the room and introduce myself and take a short history while simultaneously performing a focused physical exam. As I am doing this I will direct the nurse to obtain IV access and then administer analgesia with antiemetics. When the patient's pain has improved, I will go back and gather a more complete history and exam. In certain situations, you should not take a seat, but instead focus on multitasking for the well-being of your patient. Learn when it is that time.

CHAPTER 5
GO DIGGING IN THE DIRT

You have just finished performing a history and physical examination for your patient. You excuse yourself from the room and then sit down at your computer workstation and wonder to yourself, "Do I have all of the information that I need to go and present my patient to the attending physician?" More often than not, my guess is that you don't.

Did your patient have a recent surgery that might relate to her chief complaint today? Did you find out when the surgery was, what hospital it was performed at and who cut them open? Your patient may complain of having chest pain today. Have they had a recent stress test or a coronary angiogram? What were the results? Do they have a cardiologist? A patient presents for his third episode of syncope in the last two months. Has anyone initiated a workup to determine why this is happening?

Some patients will talk to no end and provide you with the great majority of the information you will need to put their medical mystery puzzle together. They may also provide extra information that you will need to weed through to determine if it is relevant to their ED care. Some patients may see you as an interruption of their social media surfing or game playing on their smart phone. Your presence may also be interrupting their TV viewing. No matter what the case is, it is up to you to go digging in the dirt to find out useful information.

Digging in the dirt may involve accessing old patient records through your computer or calling a patient's provider's office to have pertinent records faxed to the ED. You may need to involve a patient's family member to help you elicit additional information. In many EDs, programs that link a patient's health information together from a variety of sources are now available for healthcare providers.

If you can obtain ancillary information quickly, use it in your case presentation to the attending. If your digging might take some time, let your attending know of your plan to find the information. This will help to make you a productive provider.

CHAPTER 6
DON'T DROP THE SOAP

Congratulations! Now it's time to tell your attending about the patient you have just examined. Your presentation should use the traditional SOAP format: (S)ubjective, (O)bjective, (A)ssessment, and (P)lan. To make it even easier, I think of it like this:

(S)tuff the patient tells you
(O)bservations from your physical exam
(A)nalysis of the case
(P)roposal of what you want to do

It sounds simple enough: Retell the patient's story, report your physical exam findings, put everything together, and formulate a plan. Unfortunately, I have often heard a subjective portion that sounds something like this:

"Mr. Smith is a 54-year-old male with a past history of coronary artery disease, CHF, and diabetes who complains of a two-day history of increased shortness of breath. I hear crackles halfway up his lung fields and he has 2+ pitting edema in his legs. I think he'll need Lasix as he's got a CHF exacerbation. He denies chest pain or fever. He complains of increased swelling in his legs."

Did you catch it? The reporter put the O, A, and P in with the S. This disorganized presentation is one of my pet peeves. Say what you must say under the subjective portion and then move on to the objective findings. Over time, as your attending becomes more comfortable with you as a provider, you might be invited to report only pertinent abnormal physical exam findings. Please do your best to practice the SOAP format and respect its format in the clinical setting.

CHAPTER 7
PRACTICE YOUR PAINTING

As an eager fourth year medical student hoping to get into an emergency medicine residency program, I was rotating in an ED and trying to see as many patients as possible to impress the attending physician. I came out of the room of an elderly gentleman who was having a mild COPD exacerbation. I found the busy attending and I quickly rattled off my SOAP presentation to her. She looked at me with a tired and dull expression. She only said, "Come, sit", as she pointed to two empty chairs.

"I'm not getting a clear picture of what I'm going to walk in to see when you tell me about your patient. Is your patient older or younger than he appears? Does he smell? Is he struggling to breathe? Is he wheezing on inspiration and expiration? Whether you realize it or not, you're an artist, a painter. When you're done telling me about a patient, I should have a pretty clear picture of the patient that I'm walking in to see." She finished.

She was correct. My descriptions of the patients that I saw were drab at best. I worked on my painting throughout my residency in emergency medicine and I like to think that my artwork has improved.

Learn how to use respectful adjectives and adverbs to describe your patients and their clinical situation. "The patient looks like shit" is demeaning and you should choose different words to describe your patient's situation as you simultaneously take action to improve his status. "The patient smells like shit", however, may be correct, although the words "fecal material" would probably be preferred by many attendings. Every now and then I'm taken aback when I walk into a room to see a double amputee dwarf patient or a factory worker named Paula who used to be named Paul. I chuckle to myself in these situations and then I pull up two chairs in preparation for a talk with a junior provider about the art of painting the clinical picture.

CHAPTER 8
TIME TO GO SHOPPING

When I grew up in the 1970s, my attention was regularly drawn to an enclosed tube that sat on the living room floor and projected images onto my occipital cortex. One of these projected programs was called Star Trek and the Starship Enterprise carried a physician named Dr. Bones McCoy. At least once an episode, Bones would realize his limitations as a human and he would shout out ridiculous phrases like "I'm a doctor, not an engineer, "I'm a doctor, not an elevator", or even "I'm a doctor, not a belly dancer".

Fortunately for Dr. McCoy, he also had the help of a handheld "tricorder" that could seemingly provide an accurate diagnosis for the patient with one magic wave of the device over their body. As practitioners of medicine on Earth, there are only so many things we can garner from listening to a patient and then performing a physical exam. I can't look at you and reliably tell you your serum potassium level. Likewise, I probably can't tell you have a left bundle branch block on your EKG just by listening to your heart sounds. Luckily, we have things that can answer additional questions for us. These things are called tests. While we can use tests to find out important and timely information, the ordering of tests with a shotgun mentality of finding everything out about a situation should be avoided in all but the most critical of situations. With some exceptions, laboratory tests that won't be returned on the same day probably shouldn't be ordered through the ED. If a healthy appearing patient has a simple URI, is ordering a CBC and a chest x-ray going to change the treatment and disposition of your patient? Does the patient with lower back pain that did not result from direct trauma require x-rays? Probably not. The key words here are **clinically indicated**. Get a solid text that discusses the indications for specific test ordering in the practice of emergency medicine.

CHAPTER 9
THE GAMBLER

"You've got to know when to hold 'em, know when to fold 'em, know when to walk away and know when to run." These are inspiring words from a song called "The Gambler", made famous by Kenny Rogers in 1978. Listen to it sometime, as it's a great metaphor for life. Knowing when to hold 'em and when to fold 'em is also a big part of life in the emergency department.

As a medical student, I shadowed a remarkable emergency medicine physician and I often wondered what he was thinking when he walked out of a patient's room. Now, as an attending physician, I find myself thinking many things: "Man she was a talker", "I could sure use a coffee", and "How come the admitting doctor always calls back just when I start interviewing a new patient?" These are some of the questions I think of, but the most common question I find myself asking is "What will be the disposition of this patient?" Will I send them home or will they require hospital admission? As you become more experienced in practicing emergency medicine, you will usually get a gut feeling as to whether someone will be admitted or discharged.

Sometimes I'll walk out of a room and I won't have any great clue as to what I'll ultimately decide about the patient's disposition. I recently saw an elderly female who suffered from severe dementia. She was mildly tachypneic and had some faint crackles at her lung bases. She looked great for eighty-seven! Only when her troponin came back at 11 mg/dL and her chest x-ray showed significant CHF did I know that she needed to be admitted. Sometimes we need additional information to help our gut make disposition decisions for us.

Some providers are very conservative and admit seemingly stable patients that could probably be treated as outpatients. A very few are cavalier and would easily send home a patient with a potentially life-threatening condition. Take a guess after seeing each patient as to whether they will be admitted or not. Learn how to hold 'em or fold 'em.

CHAPTER 10
LET YOUR FINGERS DO THE WALKING

A newly hired nurse practitioner was being shown the ropes of the ED by a seasoned nurse practitioner and she was practicing her case presentations. We discussed the case of her patient who had been diagnosed with hypertension some time ago, but stated that she had wanted to attempt to lower her blood pressure through diet and exercise. The patient never got around to dieting and she didn't start exercising. A systolic blood pressure in the 190s prompted her visit to the ED.

Through testing we discovered that the patient had no acute end organ damage as a result of her untreated hypertension. When I questioned the new NP what medication she wanted to start her patient on, she said the wanted to use hydrochlorothiazide. I then questioned what dose of the medication she would start with and she looked at me intently. "I was going to look that up," was her reply. This was music to my ears and I was grinning from ear to ear.

There are going to be things that you don't know on a daily basis in the ED. Resources abound with the information you need to know. You can look things up in an app on your smart phone, a website, or, if you're feeling old school, a pocket guide or full emergency medicine text.

A busy emergency department is filled with so much noise that the last thing an attending or other provider wants to hear from someone is "What is the dose for this medication?" or "What is the phone number of the admitting resident?" or "What's being served in the cafeteria today?"

Your fingers work just as well as mine and I will look up several pieces of information over the course of a shift. Please exercise those digits to their full potential! Being able to find crucial information is a part of your job. If there is something that needs to be addressed with urgency, please ask. If you think I need to come to a room immediately to see a patient, come and get me. For the everyday stuff though, let YOUR fingers do the walking.

CHAPTER 11
A SPOONFUL OF SUGAR

In the practice of emergency medicine, we perform examinations and tests to figure out what's amiss with the human body and then we take action to fix the problems that are found. A bone is straightened, an inflamed appendix is identified, or at other times we may prescribe medications. These medications often help patients but, like it or not, they also cause many problems.

Always take the time to review your patient's medication list when you are exploring the history of their present illness. In the course of treating a patient's disease, medications may cause troublesome side effects. The patient's primary care provider may have prescribed an additional medication to combat the side effects of another. Could the medications that a person is taking be causing their current symptoms?

Take it from someone who has smacked his head at the end of a patient's workup only to then look at a patient's medication list – take a couple of minutes early in the patient's workup to check their medications. Can you measure the serum levels of any of the medications that your patient is taking? Could the reason a patient is spewing bright red blood from his rectum have something to do with the fact that his doctor prescribed not only aspirin and clodpidogrel, but warfarin too? Good bet.

Over time, you'll find your most hated medication. Mine is the rat poison warfarin. While I don't see the thousands of people going about their daily lives and living well because of this medication's anticoagulant properties, I have learned how it interacts with many different medications and causes bleeding catastrophes like few other medications.

New medications pop up on a seemingly daily basis. Watch what they're used for during your nightly TV watching or better yet, take a few minutes to research them, their mechanism of action, and their most common side effects. Beware that the cure can also harm.

CHAPTER 12
HAVE SOME DIRECTION

As a new provider, it's easy to get into a habit of seeing patients and then presenting them. You can place orders based upon what you have learned according to the patient's chief complaint. This pattern can go on for a while, but you should really try to figure out what is going on with your patient. At some point you need to develop a differential diagnosis in your head when you walk out of your patient's room.

You have not been put in the emergency department to be a robot. You are a unique provider. It is your job to do what you can to discover what is going on with your patient. The secret is that you need to have a plan to guide their journey.

I have worked with several providers who are great at going into a room to see a patient and then emerge with a boatload of patient information and physical examination findings. They are eager to tell me what tests they want to order. I will then ask them to tell me their ultimate plan for the patient, based on what they have observed. Sometimes the provider will give the blank stare of a patient having a petit mal seizure. At times, a slight head tilt will ensue, mimicking the dog who has just heard the high pitched shrill of a whistle. I'll detect a sense of stalling, as if I'm supposed to direct the provider where to go.

Your supervisor is there to check if your planned trip is appropriate, not to provide it for you. He may suggest that you alter your route to get to your goal or may even suggest you change your travel plans altogether after seeing your patient. But get a plan together, because it's one of the most important aspects of your job and you should exercise your neurons.

Take some encouragement from the late Dr. Seuss:
"You have brains in your head
You have feet in your shoes
You can steer yourself in any direction you choose.
You're on your own. And you know what you know.
And YOU are the guy who'll decide where to go."

CHAPTER 13
GET IT DONE

One of the joys of practicing emergency medicine is that you frequently get to use procedural skills to help your patients. Who else besides an emergency medicine practitioner can come home from a day's work and say that they intubated a patient, sampled another patient's cerebrospinal fluid, and put yet another's dislocated shoulder back into place? When performing procedures, you must have a knowledge of how to perform them correctly. Once you are consistently doing successful procedures, your comfort and skill with that procedure will skyrocket. There is a plethora of less commonly performed procedures that are still important in the practice of emergency medicine and these could someday help you to save a life.

I find it helpful to be able to read a concise but thorough text about a procedure before performing it. You should find a text and read it often, including reading about common procedures in your free time. For me, *Clinical Procedures in Emergency Medicine* by Drs. James Roberts and

Jerris Hedges is that text. At over 1200 pages, it is a tool to be used again and again over the tenure of your practice. You may find your own reference and should always keep it handy.

In the real world of EM, you should never be thrown into performing a procedure alone without having some level of comfort with it. Ask to observe others performing procedures early on in your training. Have a practitioner trained in a procedure by your side when you are doing it for the first couple of times. Many academic centers will have skill labs where you can practice performing procedures on cadavers. See if you can get into one of these labs.

Procedures lie at the heart of emergency medicine as a specialty. If you are doing a rotation through the ED as an elective, see and do all you can while you are there. If you will be staying a while or for a career, practice and hone your skills so that you become proficient at them.

CHAPTER 14

A PICTURE'S WORTH A THOUSAND WORDS

In emergency medicine, we often use tests to help our eyes see into the human body. X-rays, CT scans, and ultrasound studies have revolutionized the practice of EM so that we can provide definitive care for our patients that may not have even been fathomed half a century ago.

With careful consideration and experience, you will learn what radiological tests are indicated for the pathology you are seeking to find. Somewhere in a dark room, either down the hall or a continent away, a radiologist will be making money hand over fist by providing an interpretation of the tests that you have ordered. He or she will provide often verbose written reports to you of what are believed to be the significant findings of the study.

You may be tempted to accept the findings of what they have written after carefully checking the radiology report for the correct patient name. I'll urge you to resist this temptation. **Look at the films yourself first.** You have a great advantage over the physician in the dark room. You have seen and examined the patient. You know where they hurt. You know what you're expecting to see and rule in or rule out. No, you're not a radiologist, but after pairing visible radiologic images with written reports, you will become reasonably proficient at identifying common abnormalities.

There have been numerous times when I've called up a radiologist to question, "Do you want to comment on that small left sided pneumothorax on my patient?" or "Isn't that a fractured calcaneus? The patient's heel is really tender." And "I looked at the CT of the patient's head. Are you sure there isn't evidence of a small subdural hematoma along the falx?"

You have the greatest radiological cheat sheet in front of you at your disposal: the patient. If a triage nurse ordered x-rays on a patient before you saw them, examine the patient first and then look at the films. This will help you to predict where the pathology may be on your x-rays.

CHAPTER 15

GET THE LAY OF THE LAND

I magine that you're a medical or PA student and tomorrow you will be starting a month-long rotation in the emergency department. You're spending your day studying all the information that you think you'll need to answer the questions that will be asked of you tomorrow. You thought about getting off your duff and going to the hospital to check out the emergency department, but you are sure that everything will be just fine.

The next day arrives and after folding your neat white coat, you get into your car and drive to the hospital. When you get there, you discover that you can't park in the parking lot because your ID tag wasn't updated to give you access to it. After driving around, you finally find parking three blocks from the hospital. You walk through the front doors of the emergency department and explain to the greeter that you have arrived to do your rotation in emergency medicine.

The greeter calls back into the ED and ten minutes later a nurse emerges and leads you to where your preceptor for the day is supposed to be sitting. An empty chair greets you as you glance at your watch and notice it is thirty minutes past when your shift was supposed to start.

Your preceptor arrives with another student by his side. You recognize the student as one of your classmates. As they start discussing a case, they are interrupted by the nurse who gruffly announces your presence. A scowl comes over his face as he eyes his watch to subtly note your tardiness. After you introduce yourself, you feel that your preceptor has lost any good mood that he had as he points in the direction of the locker room where you are to place your belongings.

You catch the eye of your fellow student and a sly grin has come across her face. She's a go-getter and you can't help but think that she came to the ED yesterday to find her way around. You are behind in everyone's eyes because you failed to prepare yourself. Do yourself a favor and get your ducks in a row.

CHAPTER 16
WHERE'S THE THINGAMABOB?

An ambulance calls the ED over the radio. They're coming in lights and sirens with a cardiac arrest patient. He's been defibrillated twice without return of pulses. Intubation has not been attempted, but an IV line has been established. Your previous tasks are put on hold as you mentally and physically head towards the code room.

Do you know where your intubation box is? Did you check it at the beginning of your shift to make sure it was fully stocked? Where can you find a central line kit if you need it in a hurry? Has a nurse moved the code cart into the patient's room? What if the cardiac arrest patient had suffered severe blunt chest trauma but the paramedic forgot to mention that? Do you have a chest tube kit readily available?

It is very important for emergency medicine providers to know where their life saving tools are located. These are the tools that help preserve or protect the airway, breathing, and circulation. Do you know what a Word Catheter is? If it's not essential in an emergent situation, then you don't need to know where to immediately find it. However, you do need to know where to find it. Check with the nursing staff to direct you towards finding other pieces of equipment.

Early in your emergency department rotation it will be helpful to find an empty patient room and spend ten or fifteen minutes going through the cabinets in the room. Someone who can quickly find a non-rebreather mask, a Yankauer suction, a 4 x 4 piece of gauze, or IV tubing is appreciated by all the team members in the ED. Find out who is responsible for restocking the intubation boxes after they have been used. Have some down time during a rotation? Spend at least part of that time walking around to find out where things are. You'll often save yourself and your patient a good chunk of time when you are quickly able to locate supplies and equipment. As with everything in the ED, always be prepared for the unexpected.

CHAPTER 17
TELL ME NEWS I CAN USE

It was a slow morning in the rural hospital ED where I was working. I had just examined a stable patient with mild dyspnea. I entered my orders in the computer and I was about to head to the physician's call room to catch up on some reading. I asked the charge nurse to call me if anything emergent happened, assuring her that I would return to the department quickly. I settled into my chair and started reading an article whose title interested me. It had not been more than five minutes when the call room phone rang. On the other end was the nurse I had just left, informing me that my patient's chest x-ray had been completed. "Really?" I thought. I slowly walked back into the department, realizing that everyone's definition of what constituted an emergency apparently was different.

Knowing what to report and when to report it is important. As an attending physician, I am responsible for the care of all the patients in the department. Medical students seem to be the most frequent violators of the "only important news" rule. Hearing about a patient's normal sodium level and their normal hemoglobin only serves to interrupt the attention that I need to give to more important issues, especially when these updates occur at five-minute intervals. Informing me that all the tests are normal when they have all been resulted is news that I can use.

I do, however, want to hear important news and I want to hear it quickly. Knowing that Mr. Jones is seeming to be having more difficulty breathing when you checked in on him two minutes ago is important and it is something I need to go assess at his bedside. Don't be surprised if an attending physician seems aggravated with your constant reporting of normal things or your failure to report significant things. Over time, your understanding of what urgently needs to be reported will grow. Do your best to learn what is important for the immediate care of your patient.

CHAPTER 18
TIME

I t was six minutes after 7 a.m. when I hurried into the department. Not a patient was in sight and strangely, neither was a single staff member. I removed my coat and set my bag down. I headed towards the code room whose doors had been closed. I opened them to see silent nurses and my physician colleague. He had just lifted the ultrasound probe off the patient's chest and announced "Time of death, 7:08 a.m." He looked up at me and said, "Oh, good morning Dr. Borton, nice of you to join us. You won't mind writing up this poor old fellow's chart since he would have been your patient if you had been on time, will you?"

A long shift in a busy ED will beat you down, both mentally and physically. There's little worse than having to pick up a critically ill patient past the end of your shift. It's bad enough being late for shift change in a single coverage ED. When you arrive late in a teaching institution ED with many providers, your tardiness will be met with ire from a whole team that had to wait for you to sign out their patients.

I recently started working with a second-year resident in emergency medicine. He is soft spoken and clinically he's performing on a level that is on par with his fellow residents. The one thing I have noticed about him is that he is always on time. In fact, if he is coming in for the shift following mine, I know it twenty minutes ahead of time because he has arrived in the ED to check intubation boxes and to make sure that everything is ready for whatever the next twelve hours are going to throw at him.

Do whatever you need to do to make sure that you are on time (read "on time" as meaning ten minutes early) for all your shifts. If you need to, change clocks to fool yourself into being early. Weather can play a significant part in your travel time, especially in areas of the country that are prone to heavy snowfall, so plan accordingly. Being punctual will be appreciated by your colleagues, whereas chronically late arrivals will not. Respect the time of others.

CHAPTER 19
MY EYES AND MY EARS

As a provider of emergency medicine, you may be tempted to think of yourself as the most important piece in the delivery of healthcare to your patients. In a noble sense, this might be true, but realistically you are only one spoke in a complex wheel that gets things done in the ED.

Tell me how you saw thirty people during your shift without the help of nurses. Tell me how you talked to twenty different health care providers without the assistance of the department secretary. Tell me how great the flow was through your department without that housekeeper busting his or her butt all day long to clean the rooms.

The emergency department functions because there are many different people providing many different services for the ultimate care of your patients. I can't begin to tell you how many times an attentive nurse who spent a great amount of time at the patient's bedside provided me with the information I needed to pull together an unanswered question about a patient's care. Nurses are my eyes and my ears when I'm not with the patient.

A physician assistant once presented a patient to me that had reportedly come to the ED with a complaint of chest pain. The PA's story seemed a little odd for chest pain, but I instructed the provider to start a workup and I said I'd be in shortly to see the patient. When the PA left the nurses' station, a seasoned nurse pulled me aside and told me what the patient had told her. He had relayed that he had experienced weakness on his right side for forty-five minutes that had since resolved. I immediately went into the patient's room and indeed, the history he had told me was one concerning for TIA and not angina.

I consider many of the healthcare workers in the emergency department to be friends. I frequently trust their judgement and value their input. If you present a happy face to me, but you are rude or inconsiderate to other workers or patients, I'm going to hear about it. As your supervisor, I will expect you to be always treating everyone with respect, even when I'm not present. Beware...I've got eyes and ears everywhere!

CHAPTER 20
SELECTIVE SERVICE

As you spend your weeks, months, and years in the emergency department, you will get to see and treat a wide variety of patients and their pathological conditions. Over this time, you will also begin to know what maladies you enjoy treating as well as the ones you would rather pass up more than anything.

My pass up case would have to be epistaxis. Nosebleed patients are often panicked at the apparent exsanguinations that are flowing from their normal everyday air passages. Couple that with a myriad of patient medications with names like warfarin and clopidogrel, and you've got a challenge at stopping the red river that is flowing before your eyes. I will mask and gown up and use the tools at my disposal to cauterize the bleeding. I may be forced to shove an uncomfortable tamponade device up an apprehensive patient's schnoz to stop the bleeding. I HATE EPISTAXIS! It is, however, something that is encountered on a fairly regular basis in the ED and it is something that must be treated.

When I started my career, paper charts were used. These charts were placed in various bins based upon the triage nurse's assignment of acuity. I noticed one of my co-workers always picking up a stack of these charts and sifting through them. One day I questioned him as to what he was doing and he claimed that he was making sure the charts were in order of their triage time. This was happening on a frequent basis and I noticed that when I worked with this provider, I always ended up seeing messy, complicated cases. This provider's motives quickly became clear. He was chart shopping – picking up cases that he felt would be easy or desirable to treat.

Emergency medicine is full of things that you might feel uncomfortable treating. "I want to always feel comfortable" is certainly not a clause in your employment contract. Chart shopping will soon be recognized by your fellow providers and your sprees will make them resentful towards you. Do you part. Suck it up and see YOUR epistaxis.

CHAPTER 21
BECOME A MOVER OF MEAT

There are few things that can bring about a sense of dread, yet a sense of challenge, as walking into an overnight shift and seeing that there are thirty-seven patients in your waiting room just waiting to be evaluated. Sometime during dayshift, a combination of things led to gridlock. Patients that aren't moving through the department will soon become unhappy if they haven't already come to that threshold.

During a busy shift as a resident, I was falling behind. My patients had their tests completed, but I hadn't provided them with a disposition. My attending saw me sinking and pulled me aside. "What's the biggest decision you make in emergency medicine?" he asked. As my mind searched for noble and humanitarian answers, he answered for me. "It's whether to keep 'em or street 'em. Do you admit or discharge? Make that decision and then work towards that goal."

Patients may spend quite a bit of time in your department. Some of these time factors you have control over while others you do not. Here are some helpful tricks that I've learned to move patients more quickly:

- Order all the tests you'll need at one time, not one at a time
- Discharge a patient before seeing a new one
- Set forth expectations with your patients early in their stay
- Call to get a patient admitted early if they are stable
- Most discharged patients can wait for a ride in the waiting room
- Shun the ordering of non-emergent tests

These are just a few examples of how you can work to decrease length of stay in your department. With experience, you'll discover your own tricks to help move the meat in the department. Those thirty-seven patients in the waiting room will be happy that you did.

CHAPTER 22

GO TO BAT FOR YOUR PATIENT

A 22-year-old female patient had made her second presentation to the ED within a week for possible seizure-like activity. Before this, she had never had any seizures in her life. She had been seen by an attending at her first visit that had rushed her through a workup and then discharged her home to follow up with neurology as an outpatient. After her second seizure, she was rightfully scared and I cared for this patient with a quiet resident named Lisa. We had done a more thorough investigation, but we still couldn't pinpoint the reason for our patient's seizure activity.

Lisa and I talked about the case and we decided that it would be in the patient's best interest to get her admitted to the hospital to see a neurologist and get a complete workup. We found out the PMD's name and Lisa placed a call to him. This primary always hated admitting patients to the hospital and I guessed that Lisa might have a tough time convincing him of this patient's need for admission.

I was right. Lisa had done a great job of explaining the patient's situation and case, but she was still on the phone with the admitting physician after five minutes. She quietly listened to the physician's arguments and then politely countered with her own reasons as to why the patient warranted admission. I was surprised. I expected Lisa to hand the phone over to me to continue her argument for her, but she persisted.

After another five minutes of talking, I sensed a touch of anger in Lisa's voice. Finally, she blurted out, "Dr. Adams, if this was your sister, wouldn't you want her to be admitted to the hospital?" His answer must have been a "yes" as Lisa's next words were, "Great. I'll hand the phone to the nurse so you can give some admission orders."

My jaw dropped. Quiet Lisa went to bat for her patient and she wasn't going to give up until she got a hit. As an EM provider, you are the best judge of another provider's patient's immediate needs, even though the primary care provider may be very familiar with their chronic issues. Make the patient's safety your main concern no matter what.

CHAPTER 23

LIGHT A FIRE UNDER YOURSELF

There's something to be said for showing enthusiasm in emergency medicine or anything you do. As a student, an employee, or a resident, your enthusiasm will go a long way towards making you a valued provider in the ED. Your value is diminished by being a slug.

A nurse practitioner student once rotated with me who definitely could have used a good dose of epinephrine or a triple Americano coffee to get him moving. After numerous delays on his part, he finally came to do his clinical time in the ED. Within an hour of his arrival, I could see that he wasn't a go-getter at all.

When he arrived, he stated that he had not been set up with an account to use the electronic medical record. He made a couple of calls to the IT department, but by the end of his first shift, he still hadn't established an account. Throughout the day, I constantly had to prod him to get up and see patients. He did seem interested in making snide comments about the patients and working on other tasks on his personal computer. He was not interested in putting his best into his clinical rotation.

His sloth-like qualities continued throughout his rotation. He had delayed coming to the ED for his rotations during the beginning of the semester. As the time drew nearer towards the end of his rotation, he realized that he would need to work a couple of overnight shifts with me to complete his requirements. He whined about this, even though he had delayed his ED rotation as long as possible.

At the end of his last shift, he shook my hand and thanked me for being his preceptor. I was happy to see him leave. I wondered if he would last long in any job. His lack of enthusiasm triggered my lack of enthusiasm when writing comments for his evaluation. After being given fair and good marks in various areas, I simply wrote, "The student completed seventy-five hours of clinical rotation time under my supervision. He has earned a grade of satisfactory." A lack of enthusiasm on your part will serve to close doors in your future.

CHAPTER 24
THE SOOTHSAYER

Over weeks to months after starting your work in the ED, you should start to become adept at eliciting a history from and performing an exam on your patients. You will learn to order appropriate tests and when all the information is gathered, you will begin to become comfortable at developing an assessment and plan for your patient.

I think that any provider would like to get a hint that could decrease potentially hours of length of patient stays and potentially thousands of dollars in unnecessary tests. It is a simple secret that I've learned over the years and it's an easy step that usually takes less than a minute.

To perform this act of magic, head to the patient's bedside and ask a simple and straightforward question. That question should be phrased, "What brings you in today?" The question is never asked in a condescending tone. Sit down and listen to the patient. Follow your initial query with additional questions. "Oh, you called your doctor's office and they told you to come here? Who did you talk to?

Was it the doctor, the nurse, or the secretary? Were they too busy to get you in or did they think something serious was going on with you? Did you miss work today and now you need a work note? I see your brother is in the next room. Would you even be here tonight if he wasn't feeling ill?"

By asking direct questions, you will often be able to cut through any BS that may be standing between you and your patient. You might find out that your patient's doctor's new secretary was having a busy phone day and if the office nurse had been able to talk to your patient, he might not be in your ED right now for his upper respiratory infection. You will still, of course, need to elicit a careful history and perform a thorough exam.

Spending a little extra time with the patient while obtaining their history of present illness can sometimes save yourself and the patient a bunch of time by avoiding an extensive workup of a simple problem. Learn to listen to what the patient is telling you. It is sometimes helpful to ask yourself, "Could this patient have been safely managed outside of the ED?"

CHAPTER 25
BE GOOD TO YOURSELF

A verse from the Journey song "Be Good to Yourself" says "When you can't give no more, they want it all but you gotta say no, I'm turnin' off the noise that makes me crazy, lookin' back with no regrets." These are wise words for you when you work in the ED. Please remember them.

Despite our ability to help heal and sometimes even stave off death with our skills, it is important to remember that we are human and not robots. We need down time. We need time to refuel.

There is nothing that can stretch your sanity like working for twelve hours straight in the emergency department without a break for lunch or even a break to use the restroom. (Yes, I have done this more than once.)

In my opinion, you will need at least twenty minutes in a twelve-hour shift to sit down, relax, and consume fuel. Do this in a quiet break room, away from the ED so that you are not tempted to work during your break. Talk with your co-workers if you like, but not about work. Read, watch TV, or just savor the silence and your food.

Years of eating hospital cafeteria food will likely put pounds on your waistline. Make smart food choices. If possible, consider packing a homemade lunch for yourself a couple of times a week. Resist the temptation to make trips to a sugar laden vending machine.

Get up and out of your chair at work. It seems that with the dawn of the electronic medical record, practitioners spend so much of their time in front of their workstation. Go back and check in on your patients. Take a brisk walk through the department or go and empty your bladder or rectum on your employer's dime. Always make sure that someone knows that you're at lunch so that they can page you and get you back to the department in the event of a patient emergency while you are gone.

On days you are not working, engage in activities that you enjoy. Try to put work out of your mind. Spend time with friends or family. Start and continue an exercise program. Get some extra sleep and give your body the time it deserves to recoup from your work demands.

CHAPTER 26
SERVE

S hortly before his Earthly death, Jesus Christ washed all his disciples' feet. After doing this he said, "And since I, your Lord and Teacher, have washed your feet, you ought to wash each other's feet. I have given you an example to follow. Do as I have done to you. I tell you the truth, slaves are not greater than their master. Nor is the messenger more important than the one who sends the message."

Look at what one of the greatest figures in all of history has done. He performed the lowly act of washing his follower's feet. These were feet that walked through dust, mud, and dirt. They were feet that had probably stepped in animal dung. What did the leader of the greatest religion in the world do? He kneeled at his disciples' feet and washed off the dirt. He told those disciples to do the same for others.

Whether a follower of Jesus Christ or not, you can certainly learn from his example. When a patient who can eat asks you for a cup of water, be the person that gets it.

The patient will be delighted that you considered it important enough to use your time to help quench their thirst. Learn where your department keeps blankets, especially the ones in a warmer, and take an extra minute to deliver it to your patient. Nothing helps to build the trust of your patients more than showing you care about their comfort and well-being.

The emergency department can be an unfamiliar and formidable place for many. Your patients will need a pillow: get one for them. They may want the head of their bed raised or lowered: show them or a family member how to do it. They may need a urinal or a bedpan: get one for them and don't be afraid to be a servant and help them use it.

Sometimes the acuity of another patient's condition may coincide with your patient's want of a comfort need. In this case, make sure that you convey their need to someone else so their need can be met. Remember to always keep the mindset of being a humble servant while directing your patient's care.

CHAPTER 27
BECOMING A MASTER

One thousand nine hundred and seventeen. That's the number of pages in the most recent textbook of emergency medicine that I own. Two thousand seven hundred and seventy-seven is the number of pages that are in the most comprehensive textbook of emergency medicine that I own. Do I know everything in those books? Not even close. Do I know what dose of succinylcholine to give for rapid sequence intubation? 1 mg/kg. Do I know the contraindications for giving it? Yep.

Practicing emergency medicine means that you are going to learn at least a little about everything. You will determine what you need to know or it will become obvious. For things that are seen less frequently and for things less emergent, you will have time to read up on conditions and their treatments.

While it is possible to learn some of these things during your work in the emergency department, the reality in many busy emergency departments today is that you will simply not have the time to leisurely read during your shift. Know important medication doses, know ventilator settings, and know the indications and contraindications for life saving medical treatments.

For things that are encountered in your profession that you don't know about or for things that you want to know more about, write them down during your shift on a dedicated list that you keep. After your shift, or within twenty-four hours after completing your shift, spend fifteen or twenty minutes reading about each topic. Over the course of a year, you will have learned many useful things pertaining to your practice of emergency medicine.

Another way to broaden or refresh your knowledge of emergency medicine is to subscribe to a monthly subscription that offers continuing medical education credits. I use *Emergency Medicine Practice* for my continuing medical education. Always make sure that you are doing something to expand your EM knowledge.

CHAPTER 28
DISTRACTED

As I sat discussing a patient's case with a resident in the emergency department, my ears detected what sounded like the double clinking of a glass. I would have been shocked at the clinking, but with the number of clinks I had heard resonating from the PA's work station over the previous five minutes, I seriously felt I was at a wedding reception, just waiting for the bride and groom to kiss.

As I looked toward the sound of the clinking, I realized the PA had her attention and her face buried in her phone, completely oblivious to a patient's family member who was standing not five feet away from her, waiting patiently to ask her a question. When the family member had politely asked her the question, the PA gave a short and gruff answer, asking the family member to return to the patient's room. She then continued her texting party and the clinking continued for the next ten minutes.

Technology has allowed us to be in touch with our family, friends, and the world twenty-four hours a day. In the emergency department, this constant onslaught of information and communication distracts us from those who are counting on us to be present for them. They are putting their trust in us to protect their well-being.

I'm not immune to the phone temptation and I'll admit to catching up on friends' Facebook statuses at slow times during a shift. Slow times in the department may also serve as a time to catch up with friends through text messaging.

I'm suggesting a trend to moving away from this technology and more towards being there for patients. Perhaps putting a phone on vibrate or turning it completely off for three hours is not too much to ask. Briefly catch up on your need for information and communication during a bathroom or lunch break. Let your family and friends know that you're busy at work taking care of people. Being constantly distracted by your mobile device will erode your connection to your co-workers and patients.

CHAPTER 29
STARTERS OF CARE

The ambulance crew had just come through the code room door with a sixty-year-old male that suffered a cardiac arrest. He received CPR and he was intubated. An IV line was established and he was defibrillated twice. He now has a pulse and the paramedic who provided his care seems breathless as he gives report while beads of sweat drip off his forehead. His actions, as well as those of the other first responders, have saved this patient's life.

While this is a scenario that ended well for the patient, pre-hospital care providers will often arrive to the emergency department with patients who are unstable or who do not have positive outcomes. It would be easy to judge them and their care, especially when things don't go well, but a word of caution is needed before you even think about doing this.

Do you understand the local care protocols that the EMTs and paramedics follow or the limitations of care that they can provide? Did you realize that your patient is the fourth critical patient that the paramedic has cared for in the last six hours? Did you know that the EMT who is limping is doing so because she injured her knee carrying a three-hundred-pound patient down two flights of stairs? Maybe the paramedic is a bit grumpy because the pay for his job is ridiculously low and he just got off a shift from his other job that he had to take to make ends meet.

EMTs and paramedics will work their proverbial asses off to do what is best for the patient. Get to know them. Talk to them and find out who they are. Praise them when they do a good job of taking care of a patient. If you think there is a problem with their care, talk with your supervisor to determine if your complaint is something worth pursuing or if you just need a better understanding of the EMS system and its limitations. Misunderstandings can often be clarified by quietly pulling an EMS provider aside and asking them what made them do what they did. If further clarification concerning their actions is needed, report specific care concerns to your supervisor.

CHAPTER 30
TAKE NO OFFENSE

My attending physician walked out of the room where he had just interviewed a patient with shortness of breath that I had presented to him. He wore a scowl on his face. "You know what bothers the hell out of me?" he asked. "No, what?" I answered. "When a patient is hypoxic and they aren't placed on oxygen." He replied.

He was a bit perturbed with me and as we discussed the case further, he once again reminded me to supply oxygen to hypoxic patients. I've never forgotten this lesson. I'm sure this incident left his cerebral cortex long ago, but to this day, I find myself putting oxygen on hypoxic patients and putting potentially unstable patients on cardiac monitors.

The emergency department can be an extremely intense place. It may not be the best place for those who don't have thick skin. Teaching can be through questioning or it can be done through tough love. More than once I've pulled a laryngoscope out of the trembling hand of a resident who couldn't tell me the milligram per kilogram dosing of Etomidate. The next time I encountered them in an intubation setting, they knew the correct dosages for all the medications they could be using.

Don't be offended when you're yelled at or talked to sternly. This is a form of teaching that may be commonplace in your ED with certain teaching attendings. If you find that you're being yelled at for things you miss or seem to be performing incorrectly, ask if you can arrange a meeting with that physician. You may find that they may be more pleasant outside of the ED setting. You will probably learn what you need to work on for the verbal lashings by the physician to decrease in number.

Different attendings will employ different methods to help you learn the ropes in the emergency department. Learning by working with a tough preceptor is likely something you will encounter during your training or in your career. Embrace the experience, toughen your skin, and appreciate the lessons that will improve the care that your patients receive.

CHAPTER 31

THE GREAT DISAPPEARING PROVIDER

During a busy day in the emergency department, I was working with a provider who had seen three patients and had told me her plan of action for the patients she had seen. I had briefly examined two of her three patients when the nurse for the third patient came to me with a question that a family member had concerning the care of the patient.

I asked the nurse to find the initial caregiver, but she replied that she was nowhere to be found. I walked slowly through the emergency department looking for the provider and I listened for her voice at each room that I passed. My search was futile. I then called her emergency department portable phone attempting to reach her. My call went unanswered.

I went into the patient's room and performed my own examination. I was also able to answer the family member's question. Upon exiting the room, I once again attempted to call the lost provider's phone. The phone kept ringing and ringing.

I let the charge nurse know that I was walking to get a coffee and that I would return to the ED in five minutes. During my excursion, I discovered the missing provider sitting in the lobby while talking on her personal phone. I stood there briefly and heard tidbits of her phone conversation. It became obvious that her call was a personal one and not one of an emergent nature. She saw me and quickly terminated her call. I told her of my multiple attempts to reach her and of the nursing staff's inability to find her. After she apologized to me she quickly returned to the ED.

As a provider in the emergency department, you need to be available for patients and staff. If you need to leave for a short period of time, you need to inform the other providers and your immediate staff of your departure. You need to tell them briefly about any potentially unstable patients. Never become an MIA provider. It's OK to take a break at an appropriate time. Just let the right people know where you're going.

CHAPTER 32
DON'T BITCH, FIX

My patience had come to an end. After waiting for three hours for a physician to call back concerning the admission of one of his patients, I called the chief medical officer concerning the situation. For months, a group of physicians that covered each other for calls had been extremely negligent in their duty to call the ED back concerning their patients. Excuses such as "I never got a phone call" and "I'm not covering for him today" had grown stale and left a bitter taste in the mouths of most of the emergency department providers.

I explained the situation to the chief medical officer and emphasized how chronic the problem was becoming. I emphasized how patient care was suffering and how we had been asking this group to become more conscientious of their patients' needs. The CMO instructed me to admit the patient to the hospital's medical service and he assured me that he would take care of the problem.

Less than a week later, I learned that the group had surrendered their admission privileges at the hospital. Our in-house hospitalists would now be taking care of their admitted patients. When the problem had started, I complained and whined to my co-workers concerning the situation we faced with this group. It was only after I focused my energy on fixing the problem, and not complaining about it, that I saw concrete and positive results.

If your department is like most emergency departments, there are glitches and problems that need to be fixed. Focus your energy and any frustration that you might harbor towards taking positive steps to fixing the problem. Complaining makes you seem pitiful and it will only serve to bring others in the department down.

Energy used to fix problems is always appreciated, and by solving problems, you'll become a valuable part of the department. As Maya Angelou once said, "If you don't like something, change it. If you can't change it, change your attitude."

CHAPTER 33
STRAIGHT THROUGH THE DUMP

An off-service resident stood next to me during a busy shift in the emergency department, waiting to present his next patient to me. After finishing up a set of orders, I listened to him tell me how he had seen and examined an elderly female who had presented to the ED because of bright red blood coming from her rectum since awakening that morning.

After contemplating his history and physical, I noticed that he had provided no mention of the findings of the patient's rectal exam. When I questioned him about it, he replied that he hadn't performed one. He offered a poor excuse as to why the exam wasn't done as I brushed past him on my way to the patient's room. The nurse was in the room of the frail patient who looked very pale. The large amount of blood on her sheet told me she would require an aggressive resuscitation. My rectal exam revealed no palpable masses, but my glove was covered in bright red blood. A call was placed to a gastroenterologist, blood was transfused and the patient was admitted to the ICU within an hour. The resident apologized for his physical exam omission and told me he had learned a great lesson.

The practice of emergency medicine is rewarding and exciting, but it is also a dirty one. Fingers are placed into rectums and other human orifices. Contaminated wounds must be irrigated. Mucous, diarrhea, blood, and emesis are encountered daily. Malicious molecules will waft through your nares, providing you with a plethora of distinct odors you won't encounter anywhere else but in an emergency department.

Despite all of this, we sometimes having to get dirty to help our patients to the best of our abilities. Taking the often uncomfortable route will help you to find the answers that you need to properly take care of your patients. There aren't any shortcuts to take: the road to helping your patients will often take you straight through the proverbial dump. Make sure that you take the trip. Embrace the privilege that you have been given to practice emergency medicine and remember to always wash your hands before and after your trip.

CHAPTER 34
BECOME THE MAESTRO

7 a.m. sign out had just finished and our oncoming team had many loose ends to tie up from a night shift that had worked steadily for twelve hours. To my right sat an early second year resident with whom I had never worked. Her task was daunting: she had to follow up on lab and radiology tests and determine the dispositions of eight patients that had been signed out to her. She had to do all of this while picking up and managing new patients.

I envisioned myself having to work my butt off for the next three to four hours. I thought I'd be checking on lab results, calling admitting doctors and printing discharge instructions. The resident presented a couple of cases to me and after seeing the patients, I found that I fully agreed with her assessments and her plans for the patients.

I returned to my seat to document on my patients' charts and I noticed that one of the signed-out patients had been admitted and another one of them had been discharged. The resident was on the phone getting still another one of the patients admitted. As I sat there, I realized that the resident had taken the baton from me and that she had effectively become the maestro of the emergency department. I was still there for guidance, but she was, in essence, running the show.

Your ability to manage multiple patients in the ED will improve with the amount of time you spend in the department. You may push yourself to see more patients and you may fall behind, but don't be afraid to test your limits. Your supervisor will see your eagerness and should help you when you fall.

As an emergency medicine healthcare provider, one day you will walk into the department and be expected to manage multiple patients that may be critically ill. Hone your craft as you are training and learn to direct patient care to the best of your ability. Someday you will become the department maestro. Learn to skillfully test your baton throughout your training.

CHAPTER 35
EVERY PERSON TELLS A STORY

When I was a resident, I worked with an attending physician at one of the community hospitals. He taught me many disguised lessons whose value I have only now realized. He had an uncanny ability to manage a ton of patients. Patients that I had interviewed would frequently ask if he was working. He had an ability to connect with so many of his patients on a personal level. He never raised his voice and the nurses put their trust in his medical decisions without question.

After I finished residency, I joined this physician's emergency medicine group. He continued to have a great presence in the emergency department as his carried his clipboard from patient room to patient room. I'd often see him jotting down quick tidbits of information when he talked to his patients, but his clipboard never served as a wall between him and his patients.

As we sat at our desk and charted on our patients, he'd often mention interesting facts about the people he had seen. His patient with right upper quadrant pain was an accomplished woodworker. His patient with a leg laceration had recently completed her first marathon. The mother of his young patient with croup was going to return to teaching kindergarten.

He had subtly taught me another lesson. The person in room 34 wasn't just a "hot gallbladder", but a person with a story, feelings, and a life outside of their emergency department visit. By opening up to them, I could put them at ease and learn something about them as a person in the process. Both the patient and I could grow.

Neil Peart likely said it best when he penned the lines "All the world's indeed a stage, we are merely players, performers and portrayers, each another's audience outside the gilded cage" in the rock group Rush's song "Limelight". Go beyond the patient's disease and learn something about every patient you see. It will make you a better practitioner. It will make you a better human being.

CHAPTER 36

THE ART NO BOOK CAN TEACH

A ten-year-old boy was brought into the emergency department in cardiac arrest after being found unresponsive by his mother. She had last seen him well an hour before putting him down for a nap. The paramedics had arrived quickly at the house and immediately started CPR and advanced cardiac life support. They had done everything correctly. Despite their efforts, the boy never regained a pulse. In the ED, we checked and rechecked everything. Resuscitative efforts continued, but after twenty minutes, nothing changed. The patient had no pulse and no electrical cardiac activity. The bedside ultrasound revealed no cardiac wall motion. The patient was pronounced dead.

Now came the most difficult thing: Telling this patient's mother that her son who was alive just one hour earlier was now dead. I had told people that their loved ones had died before. Giving the news about older people always seemed easier for me. Telling a parent about their child's death was always devastating. I walked into the quiet room and I asked the only woman in the room, "Were you Tommy's mother?" A shocked look came over her face. I immediately realized that I should have said "are" instead of "were". My mistake haunts me to this day. I spent the next twenty minutes answering questions and comforting the mother as best as I possibly could.

As a student or a resident physician, you should go into the quiet room with an attending physician to observe how they tell a family about the loss of a loved one. You need to see how they empathize, how they act, and how they deliver the life-changing news.

As you progress, someday you'll be the one going into the quiet room to deliver bad news. Use kind words, but use direct words. Their loved one has died. I suggest bringing a trusted nurse with you to support not only the family, but also you. The nurse's experience will be a source of comfort. This part of the profession is learned only from experience.

CHAPTER 37
LET'S NOT GET TOO CEREBRAL

The emergency department can be a very busy place. Our job is to see and evaluate patients as quickly as possible and stabilize any condition that is an immediate threat to life or limb to the best of our ability. After that, we use our experience and various resources to determine our patient's pathology or lack thereof. To admit or discharge is then our ultimate decision.

I often become amused when off service rotators, particularly from internal medicine, rotate through the emergency department. They almost always perform a very thorough assessment of a patient. Then they'll report to me a plethora of information including the results of past echocardiograms and blood tests. They will likely make the decision that the patient needs to be admitted to the hospital. When I ask them what tests they want to order, for example on a patient with a CHF exacerbation, this is what

I'll usually hear, "I want to order a CMP, CBC with diff, a BNP, EKG, cardiac enzymes, chest x-ray and a PT/PTT." These are usually fine with me, but with certain providers, the list will continue. "I'd also like to get urine electrolytes, a hemoglobin A1C, and a thyroid panel…".

STOP! This is the emergency department. Urine electrolytes and a hemoglobin A1C are not going to change a single thing we are going to do for the patient in the ED. Let the admitting service order these tests for the patient. Have them put in their admission orders and get the patient to the floor.

Due to our focus, the ED is not the place to heal the whole person of all their troubles. Should we be sympathetic and listen? Yes. Should we pontificate over every non-life-threatening concern that our patient complains about during their ED visit? No, but we should be able to refer them to a reliable primary care physician who can address their long-term healthcare needs for years to come.

CHAPTER 38
FUN...IT'S ALLOWED

A local methamphetamine producer was wanted by the police for leaving the scene of a house fire that he probably ignited. His picture was plastered on the front page of the local newspaper, and as a staff nurse read it, he noticed that the wanted person's name was the same as one of the nurses who worked in our department. That part-time nurse also happened to be a full-time firefighter in the city where the meth producer had torched the house.

As I arrived in the ED for a shift, I saw copies of the newspaper article concerning the fire pinned up around the department. What had changed was that the criminal's picture had been replaced with our part-time nurse's likeness. He was due to arrive at work in thirty minutes. When he arrived, it took him about ten minutes to see the articles posted around the department. It took us another twenty minutes to stop laughing about the great prank we had pulled off.

People who work in the emergency department are usually either a little bit or way off their rocker. We are professional, but quite frequently, we are a tad bit crazy too. On the other end of the spectrum, there are those who can tramp around the department in a totally serious mood for every second of their twelve-hour shift. People come from all walks of life. If you don't think they'd appreciate being the butt of a joke, leave them alone and turn your attentions toward someone else.

The are multiple stressors in the world of emergency medicine and I believe that it is all right to laugh from time to time at work. We shouldn't laugh at the expense of our patients or their ailments, but we should be able to relax and know our co-workers as human beings who feel and laugh. That being said, we need to be mindful of the situations around us. The family that has just learned about a discovered tumor may be extremely upset at the sound of boisterous laughter emanating from the nurses' station. Let common sense be your guide as to when to have fun.

CHAPTER 39

DON'T GET POUNCED ON

The next time that your ED gets full, take a look at your tracking board. Count the number of patients you are following and see how many patients the other providers are following. Do the numbers seem consistent across the board?

Throughout my career I have observed physicians that have shoveled a fair amount of patient load on resident, nurse practitioner, and physician assistant colleagues. While a minority of these cases involve a problem with competence, the majority of these situations deal with laziness and turfing the care of the patients to others.

Every provider in the ED should be pulling their own weight, each according to their own abilities and experience. A rotating medical student in the department probably won't be able to manage six patients at a time. A seasoned physician assistant may have no problem whatsoever with caring for eight patients at a time. A new provider who recently finished an orientation process may take some time with building up their speed and confidence. There should be evidence of growth. That same "new" provider should have achieved some "developmental milestones" with their efficiency and comfort within four to six months of being at a job. Failure to do that suggests that there is a problem with the training the provider received, the provider, or possibly both.

Caregivers that are new should do the best that they can in seeing as many patients as they are comfortable seeing without becoming overly stressed. Over time, it will become evident to both you and your supervisors who is doing the job and who isn't. Providers in the ED should be given at least quarterly feedback on their level of performance. If a problem exists with a certain provider not pulling their weight, a responsible employer should provide tools to enable the practitioner to improve.

Don't complain and criticize openly. Care problems should be brought to the attention of a provider's supervisor. Don't suffer through months or years because of others who aren't working to their full potential.

CHAPTER 40

USE THE INTELLECT OF OTHERS

Let's face it; you're not the smartest person in the world. You may not even be the smartest person in your hospital, or even in the ED. In emergency medicine, you need to know a little bit about everything. There are providers who know a whole bunch more about specific medical and surgical issues that go on with your patients. Those people are called consultants.

With many patients in the emergency department, you'll get as far as you can go with their treatment and then you will be calling a consultant. Sometimes you can relay pertinent case information over the phone while speaking with the consultant and they can offer treatment recommendations without initially having to see the patient. Sometimes it will be necessary for the consultant to come to the ED to examine the patient and possibly perform a treatment or procedure. This can be a great opportunity for you to expand your intellectual horizons and learn from them.

When the consultant arrives in the ED, greet them and introduce yourself with a handshake if you haven't met them before. Get any patient information for them and show them to the patient's room. After they have seen the patient, discuss the case with them again. If they need to look at x-rays or CTs on the patient, look at the images with them. Pick their brain about a specific question you might have concerning the case. If they are going to perform a bedside procedure on the patient, ask if you can assist them or at least watch them perform the procedure. Many consultants will be happy to provide you with knowledge that may allow you to perform the procedure by yourself in the future.

When they have finished their consult in the ED, thank them for seeing your patient and for taking the time to discuss the case. If you do this every time a consultant comes to the ED, you will gain a vast amount of knowledge over the years and you will receive the respect of your consultant colleagues. Continuing medical education doesn't always happen at a conference at a tropical resort. Learn at the patient's bedside!

CHAPTER 41

HAVE SOME CONFIDENCE...

In emergency medicine, you will often be forced to make life-saving decisions in the blink of an eye without having all the information that you would ideally want to have. These decisions can sometimes make you uncomfortable. Sometimes you'll be faced with new challenges. Experience and training will help to make these decisions somewhat easier with time.

With every shift you work, patients and their families will look to you for answers and for information. They will be putting their blind trust in you to help make things better. They are expecting you to provide the best care that you possibly can. When you cannot ultimately make things better, they will look to you for words of consolation.

It will be important for you to express confidence and back up that confidence with positive results. Draw on your experience gained from previous cases and use them to build your confidence. It's quite possible that the patient you're seeing with high blood pressure, crackles on his lung exam, bilateral pitting edema, and severe respiratory distress has an acute exacerbation of his congestive heart failure. How did you treat the patient with similar symptoms last week that brought her so much relief? Can you use that knowledge to bring the same relief to the patient struggling before you with a look of impending doom in his eyes?

Express an air of quiet confidence to your patients and your co-workers. Present a plan of care for your patient with determination to those around you. There is more than one way to manage a patient's ailments and even if your plan differs from others you work with from time to time, be assured that you are doing right by your patient. Drowning in a sea of doubt about your management will only deter from your care of the patient. You have been trained to get to the point you are at today in your emergency medicine journey. Step boldly forward and let others feel comforted in your abilities.

CHAPTER 42

BUT KNOW YOUR LIMITATIONS

Hopefully I've just inspired you to race forward with confidence to slay all the pathological dragons that you will face daily in the ED. On the flip side of your confidence, you need to know when to pull back the reigns and say, "I don't know right now, but I'll find out."

On a busy evening in the ED, one of my colleagues was pulled into the room of a 42-year-old male who complained of ripping chest and back pain and he stated that he couldn't feel his left leg. My colleague stepped out of the room two minutes later stating that the patient was a "wimp" and proclaimed that there was nothing wrong with him. The concerned nurse scowled at him and muttered, "Wrong answer" as he pulled me into the room to examine the patient.

I emerged from the patient's room five minutes later and, unlike my co-worker, I was dreadfully concerned about his symptoms. The nurse and I wheeled the patient over to radiology where his CT scan revealed a large thoracic and abdominal aortic dissection with a leak. The patient died two hours later on the vascular surgeon's operating table.

In emergency medicine, you always need to keep in the back of your mind those pathological conditions that can and will kill your patients if you don't identify and treat them. With experience some of these conditions are ruled out by carefully performing a thorough history and physical examination. Other pathology will require additional tests to be ruled in or ruled out.

Remember to listen to the gut feeling that you will develop as you gain experience in the world of emergency medicine. Not every patient needs the "million-dollar workup" to rule out every emergent condition, but don't be afraid to say, "I'm not sure if this patient has this, but I'm concerned enough to order a test to see if they harbor that pathology".

In the ED, your confidence is very important for your patients. An even more important trait for your patients is your humbleness. Refuse to be cavalier in your practice of emergency medicine.

CHAPTER 43

BE PREPARED TO BE PIMPED

A prominent part of your clinical learning experience in the emergency department will likely encompass being subjected to the process of medical pimping. This is where an individual of higher clinical rank, usually an attending, will ask you a series of questions, often focusing on minute details of a medical problem, in order to force you to think on your feet.

You'll recognize when you're being pimped by that feeling of uneasiness that will emerge from your stomach. A bead of sweat might even develop on your forehead. You will search the recesses of your brain to try and come up with an answer. Some questions will probe deep into your insight of the full spectrum of a medical problem. Other questions will be asked to help the teacher discover if you know the fundamentals of emergency medicine.

Pimping can come in two forms. The first form is used to help expand your knowledge about what you know and what you don't know about emergency medicine. It is designed to help you learn. The second form may be used by an attending physician as an ego booster or to make himself appear like a god in front of others.

Pimping should never be used to make you feel personally inferior to someone else. When you are being pimped and you don't understand a question, ask your teacher for more clarification about their question. Answer the question to the best of your ability and become involved with the teaching being used. Remember to study the subject further after your clinical shift.

With time and experience, you will be able to more confidently answer the questions that you are asked. You may even begin to anticipate the questions that you will be asked concerning a patient's case. Some pimping may go beyond the relative scope of emergency medicine. Soak up the knowledge. Don't take pimping personally. It is simply a method that has been used for many years to teach people just like you in the field of medicine.

CHAPTER 44

EMBRACE THE STRANGE BIRDS

Being new in the ED can be a daunting experience. Procedures and techniques must be learned in an environment that can sometimes be hectic. Add to that a bunch of people that you've never met before with the most diverse personality traits that you'll likely ever encounter and the entire experience can seem overwhelming.

Expect to encounter people with quiet and serious demeanors to the most outspoken and craziest people you'll find anywhere on the planet. Neither of these extremes should scare you, nor should any of those personalities that fall elsewhere on the spectrum.

Years of working in an ED are bound to make anyone a tad crazy and you will quickly identify some of this craziness in your co-workers' personalities. Once these people get to know you and you get to know them, you will most likely come to appreciate their strange quirks and craziness as part of the wonderful diversity of life.

You may find that some of your other co-workers seemingly lack any sense of personality. Work to find out how to relate to them. If they are always strictly business, talk about work with them. If they seem like they don't like to talk, let it go and let them be. Don't assume their silence is due to a problem with you. Some people are naturally introverted.

Some of your co-workers may be very talkative one day and silent the next. You might want to ask them quietly if there is something you could help them with or if there is something they would like to talk about. If they chose not to talk, let them have their space. If they decide to talk to you, do your best to keep your mouth closed and your ears open. Offer only thoughtful advice to help them and don't dominate the conversation.

I encourage you to embrace the different personalities that you'll meet in the emergency department. Welcome new members to the team and remember that it once was your first day in a new and strange environment.

CHAPTER 45
DON'T MAKE ME BABYSIT

When you work in the emergency department, come to work. As an attending physician, I am here to answer your questions concerning patient care or to help direct you towards finding the answers. I am here to prevent you from harming the patient in the event that you overlook something. Think of me as your last safety gate.

You should be making a sincere effort towards moving everything else forward. Over time, you will discover how to become more efficient. You will order only necessary tests and learn the tricks to move the patient through their department stay in the most efficient manner possible.

I am not naïve. I realize that people who are new to the department including medical students, new residents, and APPs will require more supervision and they will need to be given more direction. I should also expect to see growth in a provider.

Some providers spend years in a rut of unnecessary worrying and, in the process, fail to become confident in their practice capabilities. They fret over decision making in even the simplest of cases, imagining that every single hoof beat around the corner is that of a zebra and not a horse. They seek out advice in managing nearly every single aspect of their cases.

One physician assistant I worked with in the past was very adept in managing the care of her patients. She rarely asked for guidance in their management. When she did ask for direction, she thoughtfully summed up her case and presented a very specific question as to how she should proceed in wrapping up the care. The focused questions she asked proved to me that she had carefully thought out nearly everything before coming to me.

I implore you to get feedback from your supervisors. Your employer should have at least a bi-annual evaluation process to critique your performance. Ask your supervisors to provide constructive criticism that you can use to help improve the care that your patients receive. Always look for ways to improve your confidence and value to the team.

CHAPTER 46
FORMIDABLE SURROUNDINGS

I didn't see the patient walk into the room before the medical student went in to examine him. Twenty minutes later, the student emerged and told me about the patient. I learned of his past medical history and his list of medications. I heard about his social history and his history of his present illness and his physical examination findings. The medical student then proceeded to provide a detailed differential diagnosis for the patient's chest pain. He told me that he wanted to order a barrage of tests based on the patient's past history and because of the potential for his chest pain to be something serious.

I entered the patient's room and was greeted by a man who was smiling and appeared to be in good shape. He winced in pain a bit when he coughed. When I examined him, I heard some diffuse wheezes in his lungs. I couldn't reproduce his chest pain. I asked if he had been around anyone who had been sick. His two grandsons had recently been coughing and they had paid him a visit over the past weekend. That part of the history had been previously missed.

The medical student had failed to get to the point as to why the patient was in the ED. He sought relief from the chest pain that had been caused by his cough. Even though I had hundreds of tests that I could order at my fingertips, some IM ketorolac, an albuterol treatment, and a chest x-ray were all this gentleman needed to get him on his way after his grandchild-acquired bronchitis.

As providers, we can't let our surroundings detract from figuring out why a patient is seeking treatment. Would I have sent this patient to the ED if he had presented to see me at an urgent care center with the same complaint? Absolutely not.

Can we order expensive tests to rule out life threatening illnesses? Yes, but we should perform a careful history and physical exam to make sure that these tests are warranted. The patients undergoing these tests in the ED setting should appear to be something - SICK! Learn to recognize them.

CHAPTER 47
FILTER THE NOISE

I was training a newly hired PA and we were talking about patient management when a two-year-old girl was brought into a room from front triage. The patient reportedly had increased cough and difficulty breathing over the past day. The triage nurse came out of the room and asked if I wanted to order dexamethasone. Another PA who was working that day stood up and asked me what dose of dexamethasone he should order. I suggested that he might want to go and examine the patient first. He entered the room, the nurse went back to triage, and the new hire and I continued to sit in our chairs.

"Did you see what happened there?" I asked the new PA. "No. Why, what's going on?" she replied. "Lazy medicine. Nurses making clinical judgements based on first impressions and a provider willing to accept treatment suggestions without examining the patient first. Don't get into that habit. Make your own assessment of the patient." I explained.

The working PA returned from the patient's room and questioned me as to whether or not he should give dexamethasone to the patient. He said that the patient was not wheezing and he thought that the patient had croup. I told him that I would need to examine the patient to answer his question.

I took the shadowing PA into the room. Throughout our assessment, not one barking cough was heard. We both did recognize diffuse end expiratory wheezing on the patient. The patient WAS wheezing. An albuterol nebulizer treatment and some observation showed us that the patient was improving and she was discharged to home without a steroid, but with a prescription for albuterol and a nebulizer.

As a provider of emergency medicine, there will be a large amount of noise that you will need to filter during each shift. Even though others may have years of experience with patients, make it a habit to get into your patient's room early and make your own assessment of their clinical condition. Your patients will benefit from your careful assessments.

CHAPTER 48
MIND YOUR OWN BEESWAX

A s I sat in my chair and worked on my charting, I noticed that a trio of nurses had gathered together and they were talking in hushed voices. I heard another nurse's name mentioned and then laughter ensued. Within two minutes, the nurse who they were talking about headed towards the group and they became silent as they greeted the subject of their gossip session with smiling faces.

The emergency department can unfortunately be a den of vicious gossipers who, willingly or not, may act to belittle their co-workers on a frequent basis. These acts only serve to break down the cohesion of a team that exists to help to heal and fix the human body.

Do you have a problem with a member of the staff because of something they have done or have failed to do? Take it upon yourself to pull them aside and talk about the problem. See if there is a way that the problem can be fixed simply through a better understanding of your concerns. By keeping silent and then talking to others about this person's perceived transgression, you will only make things worse for not only them, but for the entire department. Additionally, you will be perceived as a gossiper. Would you tell something confidential to someone who has a reputation of going around and talking about the latest rumor?

Elevate yourself above the temptation to become involved about gossiping about anyone. If you're in a group of people and the gossip machine starts churning, walk away. Set an example for your co-workers to follow. If you feel comfortable, defend the person being talked about and make it clear that you don't approve of the gossip that is being spread. You will be viewed as a person of integrity and you'll also be viewed as a person that can be trusted.

When you hear scathing remarks made around you, remember the words of the late Eleanor Roosevelt who said, "Great minds discuss ideas; average minds discuss events; small minds discuss people."

CHAPTER 49
HELLO MR. COMPUTER

For the most part, nearly every emergency department now employs an electronic medical record (EMR). This has led to providers needing to become fairly adept with using a computer for the input of patient information. When a patient has finally obtained a disposition, someone could review your chart and presumably see what had taken place during their time in the emergency department.

Many EMRs will include check boxes in every section of the chart, including the history of present illness section. I would strongly encourage you to either type or dictate the history of present illness section in your own words. Nothing is worse for subsequent providers than reading a series of sentences that were artificially constructed by the use of check boxes. Take the time and read one of these charts. When you do this, do you hear a robot voice in your head?

Voice dictation has helped to speed up the EMR process. If your ED has voice dictation availability, you can speak into a microphone and moments later your words will appear in the chart. Some words are picked up better than others, so take a minute to proofread your dictated words. While reviewing a colleague's previously documented record, I learned that he had identified my patient's hemorrhoids during a visit and that he had every intention of consulting these hemorrhoids for further management of the patient's condition. He had meant to say that he would consult a consultant regarding the patient's gastrointestinal bleeding.

Document everything you have done concerning patient care in the EMR. Remain neutral in your assessments, especially with patients that have displayed behavioral problems while they were under your care. Sarcastic remarks in your record will look unfavorable on your part as a provider if the patient's case ever becomes part of a litigation.

Be diligent in your charting. Learn to use approved shortcuts and templates in your EMR. Review your documentation before finalizing your work so you don't create a hemorrhoid with superhero powers!

CHAPTER 50

CONGRATULATIONS, YOU MADE IT!

You are here because you have sequentially arrived at chapter 50 or you have skipped ahead. If your arrival is because of the latter, please go back and read. Digest the advice given and fine tune it to the situations you encounter in your own emergency department. You may not yet be the great flower that you will someday become, but hopefully now you have some of the fertilizer you will need to develop strong roots in your practice of emergency medicine.

Many unnamed individuals have been provided as examples for you in this book. I sincerely thank them for showing me what behaviors and actions are helpful or not so helpful in becoming an asset for others in the emergency department. Without the enlightenment that these individuals provided over many years, my words of advice in this book would not have been possible.

It is my wish that you find great joy in providing emergency medical care for those that you signed up to serve. Your calling will sometimes push you to your mental and physical limits. You will experience days when you ask yourself why you ever came down this career path. This is perfectly normal. Your moments of doubt will be countered with great victories... a painful dislocation is reduced; pain is alleviated; your careful suturing starts to heal broken skin; you make the unstable patient stable again through the work of your mind and hands as your quick actions restore life to another human being.

You will serve thousands and thousands of people throughout your career in emergency medicine. Remember that you can learn something from every one of them. Use the tools that you have been given to become a better provider with each passing shift. Expand your knowledge through reading and hands on learning. Remember that in order to help others, you also need to take care of yourself. Take time to rest and experience life away from the world of emergency medicine. Thank you for reading this book. May you practice the ABCs of making it in the ED!

Made in the USA
Columbia, SC
16 January 2020